The Paleolithic Diet

What It Is and Why It Works

By Mackenzie Jagger

http://theflatbellysolution.org

Other Books
By
Mackenzie Jagger

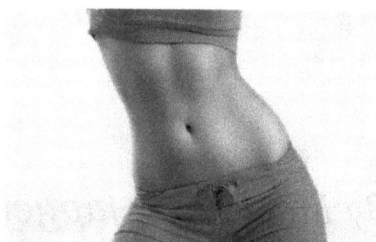

Mackenzie Jagger

THE
BELLY FAT
DIET BOOK

Why The Flat Belly Diet is The
Ultimate Plan for Melting Belly Fat

This book is dedicated to all those who have struggled to eat healthily and maintain a modest weight.

May this book be a new beginning for you!

To Your Success!

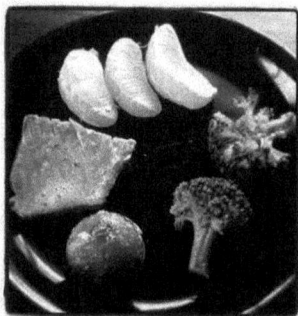

The Paleolithic Diet is NOT a fad. It is the diet that was eaten by our ancestors, the Paleolithic humans around 2.5 million years ago. Research has revealed that the diseases that afflict the modern societies today were not present during the Paleolithic age.

Inside "The Paleolithic Diet - What it is and Why it Works" Mackenzie Jagger explains why following this caveman diet book results in benefits we all are striving to attain and why this diet has had a resurgence like no other diet in history.

She answers the question "Is the Paleo Diet for Athletes?" and although this is not specifically a Paleo Cookbook, Mackenzie includes Paleo meal plans for every meal from breakfast to dinner with snacks and desserts as well. You're bound to become a healthier person just because of its nutrient rich nature. Just wait till you see some of these caveman diet recipes.

Yes, I'm sure you'll agree that paleo nutrition is built into everything you'll eat and Mackenzie gives you the one question you'll need to ask yourself before you decide whether you should eat a particular food or not. And once you know what foods you can eat you'll be creating your own personal Paleo Recipes in no time!

The positive nutritional value is going to exist in anything you eat within the program, so let's make it fun! Omelets, soups, salads, stir-fry, and even chicken Marsala are all delicious options for the Paleolithic dieter, and it does not stop there!

I don't know whether or not the Paleolithic diet is the solution for you or not, but... why not give it a chance?

Let's get started!

Table of Contents

Introduction - What is the Paleolithic Diet?   1

Does the Paleolithic Diet Work?   9

Paleolithic Diet Weight Loss   13

Getting Started with the Paleolithic Diet   17

    Approved Paleolithic Diet foods

Paleolithic Nutrition   21

Paleolithic Diet Breakfast Ideas   27

    Southern California Omelets

    Poached Eggs with Salsa

    Scrambled Eggs with Basil & Scallions

    Quiche Recipe

Paleolithic Diet Lunch Plans   35

    Roasted Chicken Salad

    Chicken & Lettuce Wraps

    Chicken, Vegetable & Mushroom Stir-Fry

Paleolithic Diet Dinner Plans   41

    Steak & Mushrooms, with a Side Spinach Salad

    Grilled or Baked Fish & Vegetables

    Lemon & Garlic Scallops (or Shrimp!)

    Grass-Fed Beef

Paleolithic Diet Desserts   49

Paleolithic Diet Snacks   51

Paleolithic Diet Support   53

Paleo Diet for Athletes   57

       Breakfast or Pre-race Meal Ideas

       Lunch or Short Term Meal Option

       Dinner or Long Term Meal Option

Closing Thoughts   65

Recommended Reads   69

About the Author   71

Disclaimer   73

Introduction

What is the Paleolithic Diet?

THE PALEOLITHIC DIET, WHICH IS also referred to as the Hunter-gather Diet, the Caveman Diet and the Paleo Diet, is a nutritional plan that dates back to its namesake ancestral period of the Paleolithic era. This lengthy era began approximately 2.5 million years ago, and only ended around 10,000 years ago with the advent of agricultural growth opportunities; namely the addition of grains.

Simply put, before our ancestors could partake in the unhealthy grains, legumes, dairy, refined salt and sugar and processed foods and oils, they were left with a healthy meal of fish, seafood, grass-fed, free range lean meats, eggs, fruits, vegetables, nuts, fungi and roots. This diet afforded them, much like it will you, a healthy digestive system, unencumbered by processed foods.

When you think of the diet in dated terms, it is simply the procuring and preparation of foods that existed during that time frame, in a natural way. Since there was no such thing as butter, they would use coconut oil, or oils from natural seeds and nuts. Instead of using refined, hard to process sugars, they would use honey, or a similar natural sweetener including flowers or sprigs. Ideally, whatever they could hunt and gather naturally was their standard diet. In modern day terms, that means no processed or packaged foods. It means no immune repressing additives that lead to illnesses, bloating and obesity.

This substitution is a great thing, mostly because it requires dieters who adapt its genius to think about what they eat before they purchase it, and consume it. The next time you go for an already prepared meal, consider its contents and ask yourself if this was something your ancestors would have eaten. Probably not. Since potatoes and grains were not a part of their agricultural make-up then, you too will have to say goodbye to them, and that is a fantastic thing for your health and happiness.

What's more is that researchers believe that the human body has changed very little from the Paleolithic era, which means subsisting on the foods that were available during that time is still ideal to the human digestive system. In fact, medical professionals agree that following the Paleolithic Diet has a track record of delivering individuals from the risk of heart disease, obesity, hypertension, Diabetes, gout and allergies.

It shouldn't be a surprise that a lot of human health problems begin with what we eat. Amazingly, people understand that they cannot feed their pets greasy, processed foods, lest they become ill, and their digestion be interrupted in a negative way. However, they will ingest the exact same meal that is not fit for their dog to eat, and expect it to process in a different manner. It doesn't. Fatty, processed, high sodium or sugary foods process slowly, and upset the gastrointestinal system along the way, no matter who you are.

Luckily, in the modern world, the Paleolithic Diet is easy to accommodate, as most people have access to fresh food without issue. In the Caveman days, it was certainly necessary for each person and their family to hunt and gather foods that were readily available in their region. In some cases, they would have to go on hunting or fishing excursions simply to capture a large amount of protein for their families to live and eat happily and healthily.

Now days, you can simply head to your favorite market and pick up fish or seafood, cucumbers and mushrooms, delivering a perfect Paleolithic Diet meal in a matter of minutes. With all of the fresh meats, vegetables and fruits available these days -- in grocery stores, specialty shops, farmer's markets and even restaurants, there has never been a better time to adapt to the Paleolithic Diet lifestyle.

In the same vain as the food choices available in the Paleolithic Diet, which do not include any fructose-laden options, alcohol, sodas, fruit juices and fermented beverages are also off the table. Water is a perfectly suitable hydration source for this diet, and its increased consumption will only provide benefits to the appearance of your skin, hair, and internal organ operation. In addition, Coconut Water has become wildly popular in many markets, and is a delicious approved beverage for this diet.

Lastly, foods in this diet can be cooked to your heart's desire, so your entire family can participate in some form of its initiation. It is not the same as the "Raw Food Diet" where everything you eat is uncooked. You can cook the fish, seafood, meats, eggs and vegetables to your liking, as long as you are not adding butters, sauces or cheese to them during the process. Remember, the diet is based around items that actually existed before the Neolithic agricultural revolution.

Researchers and medical professionals agree that there is a ratio of consumption involved in the success of this diet, so simply eating lean, grass fed beef each day for the duration of your diet may not provide the results you were hoping for.

Instead, 55-65% of your diet should be derived from animal foods, with the balance coming from plant foods. Although it is not exactly half and half, the basis is set for an even distribution of your energy sources.

This diet can deliver anyone who chooses it from

the weight inducing processed foods that account for 70% of the food energy humans devour each day. Processed foods, dairy, grains, salt and refined sugars and vegetable oils are all contributors to the industrial illnesses of obesity, heart disease and diabetes.

Does the Paleolithic Diet Work?

The short answer is yes, and here is why. When you are following a diet that is high in protein and plant consumption, you are ingesting micronutrients that transfer to digestible energy. This means your body does not have to work as hard to create energy from the sustenance you consume.

Unlike grains and dairy, which take longer to process, thereby slowing down your metabolism and your energy sources' output altogether, this diet works with your body's natural digestion and energy processes.

9

What's more is that the Paleolithic Diet components are higher in vitamins, minerals and nutrients than their processed or agriculturally acquired counterparts. The Paleolithic Diet is successful in delivering micronutrients that are hard to come by in other foods, including omega-3 fatty acids, iron, zinc, copper, iodine and selenium, which are essential to brain development and function.

A Paleolithic inspired diet not only works for weight loss purposes, but it is also exceptionally beneficial to your digestive and muscular health. With the lack of processed and modern day foods, you will experience less bloating, and a state of regularity that is healthy and natural to your body's everyday routine. Likewise, you will be able to build more muscle, and keep it healthier, longer throughout your consumption of the ideal Paleolithic Diet foods making it an excellent diet for athletes.

The Paleolithic Diet is your first defense against disease and obesity, and should be enjoyed by picking foods that you already love that fit into the approved categories. Consider the parameters of the diet, and begin making a list of all the foods you love that fall into the Paleolithic Diet classifications of consumption. This will help you create a realistic plan for proceeding with the diet.

As all dieters are aware, being realistic about your options is the cornerstone of success in this arena. Unrealistic restrictions are another reason why a lot of other diets fail. Eating only cabbage or kale, or ingesting only liquids for an entire week is unhealthy and unrealistic! If you cannot stick the program, because it is so outlandish, why even try?

The minute someone abandons a diet they begin to feel as if they have failed. This is a slippery slope, and usually results in a binge of some sort, whether it is food or alcohol. Neither alternative nor sulking tactic is recommended for any reason, so do not set yourself up to fail. Be smart in your nutritional intake, and try something that people have longed developed as a healthy plan to health and weight loss.

Paleolithic Diet Weight Loss

Weight loss is going to come fast and furiously with this diet, simply by excluding the items that do not fall within the Paleolithic dieting efforts. Assuming you have to toss anything that is in your home or office that is in a package, processed, pasteurized dairy and, of course, junk food, you are already providing yourself with a healthy alternative to cravings.

If the unhealthy options are not available, you cannot consume them! If you cannot consume them, you are not ingesting empty, non-essential foods to your system. It's a great start, and one that will get you far in your weight loss efforts.

Likewise, since the Hunter-gatherers did not own deep fryers, or vegetable oils, you can omit those items from your diet as well, which means stopping at a drive-thru is no longer an option. If you counted on a cheeseburger value meal - containing a cheeseburger, fries and a soda -- from your favorite drive thru as a meal option even once a week, this diet just saved you 910 calories, 31 grams of fat, 8.5 grams of saturated fat, 1.5 grams of trans-fat, 890 milligrams of sodium and 40 milligrams of bad cholesterol.

If you ate there more than once a week, or fed your family a similar meal more than once in any given week, you do the math. Although it may be saving time, it certainly isn't adding anything positive to your diet or nutritional intake. If anything, it is providing the exact opposite effects, which can be incredibly harmful to your overall health.

Now consider all of the other things you consume throughout the week that do not fit into the healthy Paleolithic diet plan.

This assessment is not necessarily to beat yourself up about the energy choices you make each day. It is simply necessary to honestly assess your current eating habits in an effort to replace them with healthy, protein and vitamin rich alternatives that you enjoy, so weight loss becomes effortless. When dieting becomes a chore, practitioners abandon the process, which means they are not getting healthier or losing weight. The Paleolithic Diet provides its users with real time solutions to weight loss that work, and gives them a healthy constitution as a result.

Getting Started with the Paleolithic Diet

The first step in preparing for the Paleolithic Diet is to have an opened mind about the process, and how it will affect your health. You are going to become leaner, healthier and more positive as the diet continues to work, and before you know it you will be eating new foods and enjoying life at an accelerated pace.

Approved Paleolithic Diet foods include:

- Fish -- any kind, from any natural water source

- Seafood -- any kind, from any natural water source

• Lean, Grass-fed Meats -- range free chickens and beef

• Free Range, Organic Eggs

• Vegetables -- If you can eat it raw, it is approved. That means beans, grains and starch based vegetables are out

• Fruits -- Fresh fruits only, no juices or dried versions

• Nuts and Seeds -- Unsalted, natural nut and seed sources of almonds, macadamias and pistachios or sunflower seeds are all great sources, but should be limited to four ounces per day.

PEANUTS ARE NOT ALLOWED –
THEY ARE CONSIDERED A LEGUME.

• Oils -- Olive, coconut and nut oils are all approved, but should be used sparingly.

• Hydration -- Water, water and more water. Organic, caffeine free teas are also approved for use, but should not be drowned with processed sweeteners. Coconut water is also a great source of hydration, and is available just about everywhere, even if you don't live on an island!

If it is simply not realistic for you to cut your entire meal intake into the above categories, due to family or financial restraints, or simply because you think you will fail immediately, start the process in stages.

Stages can include slowly eliminating cheeses or dairy products, so you are only eating them once or twice a week, and not with every meal. Likewise, consider changing your salad dressing to a balsamic or red wine vinegar to get you started in the right direction. Try using spray cooking oils instead of butter, before switching directly to the better oils.

If free range meats are out of the question, consider using leaner cuts of chicken, beef and ground beef. If at all possible, purchase these items from a butcher or deli, instead of the packaged versions that are prepared in Styrofoam bottomed containers.

In addition, you can use canned tuna and salmon as replacements where fiscally necessary. The choices in your meal preparation are also deciding factors, so don't beat yourself up if you cannot afford to purchase all of your meats from a local market at first.

You will slowly be able to incorporate the necessary items as the diet moves along, so if you need to start out slow, please do. Again, the goal is to succeed in this lifestyle, not abandon everything at once and regret it immediately.

Think logically where this diet is concerned, and adapt it to your lifestyle with the absolute goal of being committed to the Paleolithic Diet sooner than later.

Paleolithic Nutrition

When you consider the approved food options, begin making lists of what you love about its composition. For most, eggs and fish become a very steady part of their diet, and can be consumed in any variation they choose -- as long as it is naturally prepared.

This diet and its nutritional content can be very easy to adapt to by using this one clear question: Could a Caveman (or woman) have eaten this? If so, proceed with it in your diet!

The positive nutritional value is going to exist in anything you eat within the program, so make it fun! Omelets, soups, salads, stir-fry, and even chicken Marsala are all delicious options for the Paleolithic dieter, and it does not stop there!

Once you discover the nutrient rich foods you have always liked, including a lean cut of beef cooked or rare, with a side of mushrooms, onions and bell peppers, with sliced red tomatoes on the side, you will enjoy each meal with open arms.

When you are ready, and there is certainly no pressure, you can start trying foods you have never eaten. This diet opens up a whole new, delicious world of nutritional options, with items that the everyday person may not even know they like!

Items like:
- Zucchini
- Eggplant

- Spinach
- Kale
- Avocado
- Wild Mushrooms
- Cantaloupe
- Berries (blue, black and raspberry)

In addition, this diet will help you discover new ways to season your food without salt, butter or preservatives, starting with all of the delicious spice staples a person could dream of. This segment of the diet can be adopted immediately, no matter what level you are working towards. Get rid of the salt and butter altogether, and concentrate on spices and herbs for flavor.

- Oregano
- Basil
- Black Pepper
- Parsley
- Garlic
- Cilantro
- Cayenne Pepper

- Paprika
- Dill
- Tarragon
- Thyme
- Rosemary
- Sage
- Cumin
- Mint
- Cinnamon
- Fresh Juice from a Lime and Lemon
- Olive, Flax & Coconut Seed Oils

These allowances mean you can bake a delicious piece of fish in the oven or on the grille with a teaspoon of olive oil, a lovely douse of dill or basil, and the squeeze of a fresh lemon, while you bask in the fact that it is, absolutely, considered a diet.

Not only are the approved foods delicious options, but they are good for you and your family!

A key component to this diet's success is eating

foods that you enjoy. Do not try and cram your meals with spinach and zucchini if you do not enjoy how they taste. Simply stick to romaine lettuce and tomatoes instead if those are things you enjoy.

Likewise, find spices that you enjoy and incorporate them into your meals. In fact, once you are familiar with the herbs and spices that you like most, consider growing your own. There are a number of starter kits available at your local home and garden retailers, and they are designed to fit into your window sills easily, so there aren't any space-related issues that come along with growing your own herbs.

In addition, they can be grown year round, since they are inside, and make an amazing addition to any meal. Plus, they are incredibly fragrant and look beautiful as they grow, so it is a win/win/win!

To help get you started in the right direction, here are a few meal ideas, starting with breakfast, and getting you through to an evening snack. Keep in mind that this diet does not involve you cutting down on your meal intake, but simply the idea of introducing smart, Paleolithic alternatives when you do eat.

Paleolithic Diet Breakfast Ideas

If you are a fan of eggs, you have picked the right diet! The Paleolithic Diet gives you free reign in the free range, *organic* egg department. You can eat them poached, scrambled, in omelets and hard boiled any time of day. Here are a few fun combinations to make breakfast one of your happiest meals of the day.

Southern California Omelets

Here's a hint, and something you will learn as your avocado consumption increases: Anything considered "Southern California Style" simply includes the Super Food's participation in its preparation. This beautiful omelet isn't any different, and it packs a great punch for getting your day started.

Whisk three free range, *organic* eggs into a bowl while you prepare a pan with a tablespoon of extra virgin olive oil, heating it accordingly. Add the eggs to the pan until they are nearly cooked throughout.

Add one cup of chopped spinach to one side of the omelet, seasoning with basil and black pepper for taste, and fold the omelet in half. Place the omelet on a plate, add the equivalent of one small avocado to the top in slices, and enjoy the delicious combination!

Poached Eggs with Salsa

First things first, this diet is the perfect catalyst for an addition to your cooking tools. To enjoy your egging options to their fullest extent, you are going to need an egg poacher. It is a simple, metal contraption that you can crack eggs into to cook them in a healthy manner over boiling water. They are available at just about any big box retailer, or kitchen and bath store, and are simply fantastic to have around to increase your egg preparation variety.

In the case of poached eggs and salsa, simply prepare the poacher by greasing the side walls with flaxseed or olive oil. Place the poacher over boiling water and add the eggs. Allow them to cook for 6-7 minutes to insure they are poached to perfection. Transfer the eggs from the pan to a plate where you will add a delicious salsa atop, which you can prepare ahead of time.

To make a perfect salsa, use one cup of peeled and chopped tomatoes, add one quarter cup of chopped red onions, one quarter cup of green or yellow bell peppers, one tablespoon of lime juice, two teaspoons of cilantro, and cayenne pepper to taste.

Spoon the salsa on top of the eggs in any quantity you wish. You can use the entire serving if you would like! In addition, you can substitute the tomatoes for peaches or grapefruits to add a tangy addition to your poached perfection!

Scrambled Eggs with Basil & Scallions

One very delicious breakfast option comes in the simple form of four ingredients: Extra Virgin Olive Oil, Eggs, Basil and Scallions. Whisk three eggs into a bowl, adding a pinch of basil (and black or red pepper, if you feel spicy!) and finely cut scallions in at the same time. Heat a pan with a tablespoon of extra virgin olive oil on the stove, and add the mixture to the pan.

Allow the eggs to cook half-way through before scrambling them to perfection. This entire process takes approximately five minutes to accomplish, and the energy you will receive as a result will last well into your lunch hour.

If you are in an even bigger hurry in the morning, you can settle for one of the following, easy to grab and go options:

- Berries & Coconut Milk
- Mixed Nuts, Seeds & Berries
- Grapefruit, Peach or Fruit of Your Choice
- Coconut Milk & Fruit Smoothie
- Hard Boiled Eggs
- Prepared Quiche

Preparing quiche ahead of time is a great idea, as it allows you to grab a meal on the go, or simply settle into your evening a little easier after a long day at the office by slicing off a portion and heating it up for an easy meal. The Caveman may not have had microwaves, but we do -- and they are a great source of heat, so take advantage of it!

You can also cook the scrambled egg recipe in a

microwave safe bowl to avoid using the stove at all in the mornings!

Quiche Recipe

In a 9" x 9" pan, grease the sides and bottom with a flaxseed or extra virgin olive oil and set it aside. In a bowl, stir eight large, free range organic eggs to frothy consistency and add one whole chopped yellow onion, and ten ounces of chopped spinach (washed thoroughly, of course).

Add red and black pepper to taste, along with any other herb you enjoy. Pour the mixture into the oiled pan, and place in a pre-heated oven of 350 degrees. Allow to cook for 30 minutes, or until a toothpick can be inserted into the middle of the quiche and be removed cleanly.

Allow to sit for ten minutes before serving, or refrigerate the whole pan for later meals. This will feed one or two people for several mornings, lunches or evenings.

Breakfast is pretty easy, because eggs have such a heavy use in the mornings. However, do not be afraid to mix it up and have eggs for lunch or dinner. You do not want to get burnt out of one of the best components of this diet too quickly, so be sure and use your versatility in preparation to keep your interest up.

Paleolithic Diet Lunch Plans

Since salads, vegetables and fruits are going to be a large part of your daily meals, start thinking about all of the things you love and consider mixing them together. For instance, adding grapefruit portions and almonds to a spinach salad makes a perfectly sweet and salty combination that everyone craves from time to time.

Here are a few additional ideas to keep your lunches exciting and delicious.

MEAL PREPARATION TIP: When you are preparing meats in your home, make a lot of them. For instance, if you are going to prepare a chicken, prepare a whole, free range organic chicken in the oven. Simply wash it thoroughly and rub it down with your favorite spices before cooking it using the directions provided.

This allows you to make salads, wraps and quick grab protein ideas with already prepared foods, so you will not have to cook a chicken breast every time you want to add it to the salad. Simply clean the bird of its meat once it is cooked, store it in a sealed bowl or bag for use throughout the week, and toss the bones and skin immediately.

To enjoy it immediately after cooking, simply team it with a delicious steamed vegetable of your choice, and a fruit salad to add a bit of acidity and sweetness to the meal.

Roasted Chicken Salad

Here's your first chance to use the chicken's leftovers!

Grab a large bowl from your cabinet and fill it with the leafy greens of your choice. Romaine, spinach, kale, you name it -- toss it in. Add tomatoes, carrots, red onions, red, green or yellow bell peppers, and mushrooms, along with shredded chicken that you have already prepared.

Top the salad with a combination of lemon juice, extra virgin olive oil, and black pepper and serve garnished with avocado or fruit of your choice. Eat the entire bowl, if you'd like! One great tip for meal preparation using the Paleolithic Diet is to make it as colorful as possible!

Enjoy a variety of colors in everything you cook by adding different vegetables and spices. Everyone loves a beautiful meal!

Chicken & Lettuce Wraps

Option number two for that perfectly roasted chicken hanging around your fridge... Add the shredded chicken to leaves of lettuce, toss sliced almonds atop the combination, and add a dash of rosemary and lemon zest to the top before folding and eating. This fresh concoction is perfect for a quick and savory meal and can be prepared ahead of time, if necessary.

It's perfect for brown bag lunches, or for placing in a cooler for a picnic. The ingredients cannot get too cold, eating them directly from the refrigerator is an awesome, low maintenance alternative to processed meats and cheeses.

Chicken, Vegetable & Mushroom Stir-Fry

The best thing about stir fried meals is that you can toss in any approved foods you would like, and use all of the spice combinations that make you happy without worrying about blowing your diet. Simply toss fresh bell peppers, mushrooms, cherry tomatoes and chicken into a pan with a tablespoon of extra virgin olive oil until cooked thoroughly, and enjoy it with chopsticks from a bowl.

The bowl will help keep the ingredients warmer, longer. The chopsticks are just a fun alternative to a fork! You can also substitute fresh fish, seafood or beef as a substitute for the chicken in both of these cases, to add a little variety to your salads and stir fry.

Paleolithic Diet Dinner Plans

The best helpful hint applies to dinner, even more so than any other meal: *Cook a lot of food at dinner, and eat the leftovers during breakfast and lunch.*

Imagine tossing a bit of leftover beef into your omelet the next day, or adding it to your quiche (meat should always be cooked before placing it in a quiche recipe -- never expect raw meat to cook within the egg mixture).

Likewise, it makes for a perfect protein option for upcoming meals, without going through the cooking process all over again.

Steak & Mushrooms, with a Side Spinach Salad

This perfectly delicious and healthy meal gives you every option to prepare a meal to your exact specifications, even if you are preparing it for two people, or your entire family.

First, your steak can be prepared to your exact liking, temperature wise, but it can also include spices that the other person's does not.

So, go ahead and rub your steak with cracked pepper before you prepare it, and eat it as rare as you would like! Just throw on everyone else's cut beforehand, so the meal is ready at the same time. This is how you currently operate when grilling, so nothing changes.

In addition, drop as many mushrooms as you can eat into a sauté pan with a couple drips of extra virgin olive oil and toss them around until they are hot. Toss a handful of spinach into a bowl with a tablespoon of almond slices and the squeeze of a lemon wedge, and you will be feeling refreshed by your incredible meal, without feeling full and weighed down.

That is the beauty of the Paleolithic Diet. You will not feel like you need to take a nap after you eat, but instead will be ready to take on the evening's events with fervor and energy.

Grilled or Baked Fish & Vegetables

If you were never big on eating fish before, you may need to go through a few different types to decide which ones work best for you. Mild, white fish is the best way to go initially, as it provides a great introduction to how fish cooks and tastes as a result. Then you can move on to the beautifully flavorful options of tuna, salmon and rainbow trout.

Whichever you choose, you can easily prepare the fish by cooking it in a tablespoon of extra virgin olive oil, and seasoning it with your choice of basil or dill, and fresh crushed garlic, with a splash of fresh lemon juice during the cooking process and after it has been plated.

In addition, steam the vegetables of your choice as a side, or slice a large tomato and lace it with cracked black pepper.

Lemon & Garlic Scallops (or Shrimp!)

Scallops are a beautiful meal, all by themselves. Add steamed or stir fried zucchini strips as a side, and you have the perfect meal any day of the week.

Simply heat a frying pan with a tablespoon of extra virgin olive oil, and toss the scallops, fresh crushed garlic, and finely sliced white onion into the pan and cook until hot. The scallops can be cut in half to ensure their ideal temperature is reached, and that you are not eating uncooked seafood. They will become firm and browned on the outside when cooked thoroughly.

Squeeze fresh lemon juice over the whole pan during the cooking process, and again after it is plated. Toss the zucchini into the pan when you are drawing close to the scallops' completion, so the strips are simply heated and served al dente. You can substitute shrimp and bell peppers in place of the scallops and zucchini, as well, cooking each the same way.

Grass-Fed Beef

When you are shopping at your local butcher or in your grocery's meat department, look for grass-fed beef to prepare in large quantities. It could be in the form of a roast, or larger cuts of beef that you can prepare at once and use later in the week to add to your breakfast, lunch and dinner options.

It also helps provide you with a variety of ready to eat foods throughout the week, so never be afraid to cook too much food. With this diet it isn't the amount of food you eat, it's the variety of food you eat.

So grab a large roast, and enjoy it throughout the week with your poached eggs, in a salad, or as a meal with your veggies and fruits. Also, do not be afraid to sit down with a giant, grass-fed steak one evening and enjoy it all by itself! This is one of our favorite meals, as it gives us the gluttonous feeling we long for at times, while still maintaining our approved diet.

The following meal, we promise ourselves, will be all veggies and fruits. It is a nice way to mix up the balance, and a perfect way to enjoy just one segment of the diet, instead of the constant incorporation during most meals.

Mix it up and enjoy the options you are able to eat, with every day that passes. They are all delicious, and can be eaten at your local restaurants as well, so you will not have to eat like a crazed dieter when you are enjoying a business luncheon or dinner with clients.

Menus, thankfully, are evolving to include organic food options that were not available before, so no one will even need to know that you are "dieting"! You will simply be eating a delicious, healthy meal from the menu.

Speaking of not "dieting", there are a number of awesome dessert options available in the Paleolithic Diet platform as well, which really helps those with a sweet tooth get by during the first stages of the diet

Paleolithic Diet Desserts

One of the worst things about a standard diet is that desserts are out -- no matter what you consider as a treat. This is not so with the Paleolithic Diet. Sure, you can't eat a giant serving of processed and packaged cheesecake, but at this juncture in your life, why would you even want to?

Instead, try these fanciful delights on for size, and maintain yours in the process!

- Baked Apples
- Coconut Ice Cream
- Poached Port Wine Pears
- Cherry & Berry Medley Mix
- Fruit & Nut Medley Mix

Paleolithic Diet Snacks

Dieting snacks have never been easy to come by, but with the Paleolithic Diet all you have to do is consider the approved foods, and prepare your snacking options around them.

- Nuts & Seeds
- Sliced Vegetables, including Celery, Bell Peppers & Cherry Tomatoes
- Whole Fruits, including Apples, Peaches, Oranges & Grapefruit
- Homemade or Organically Crafted Beef Jerky
- Hard boiled Eggs
- Mixed Berries

Paleolithic Diet Support

Although the Paleolithic Diet is considered more of a lifestyle than an actual diet, it is going to be important that you stick to the healthy eating plan by discussing your approved foods with your friends and family, to garner support throughout your weight loss journey.

If nothing else, they may be able to provide you with awesome food preparation ideas to mix up your meals! In addition, you just might inspire someone else in your social group to take the first step in improving their health.

If you would rather keep your new lifestyle to yourself, in an effect to avoid any saboteurs along the way (yes, they exist, and you probably already know that), there is an entire network of online support groups, forums and healthy eating guides that can help you stay the course.

The overall benefit of the Paleolithic Diet is the improvement of your overall health, which includes weight loss as a side effect. You are going to become thinner, healthier, and have more energy than ever before, which will allow you to participate in more social and physical activities that will contribute to enhancing your healthy lifestyle.

It is important, however, that you enjoy the journey. It is important to love the foods you eat, and keep an eye out for anything unnatural -- no matter how well it is disguised otherwise.

Do not be afraid to read labels when foods have them, and to pick up only fresh items when they are available. You will get the hang of it rather quickly, and will find that your shopping list remains pretty consistent from week to week, so there will be fewer surprises as your new lifestyle evolves.

Paleo Diet for Athletes

Bending the Rules for Training, Exercising and Recovery

The one segment of the Paleolithic Diet that will differ for a single group of people is the adaptation of the Paleolithic Diet by athletes. Athletes can benefit from the diet's cleanliness in the same way that everyone else does, but because they are inherently using more calories and energy with each workout, they must consume carbohydrates to keep up with their output.

In addition, athletes need to eat before, during and after extended workouts to insure that their bodies are nourished according to their physical output. That means incorporating sports drinks and starch into their diets. Keep in mind the following sample menu is for endurance athletes who run, bike and perform at a competitive level.

Breakfast or Pre-race Meal Ideas

Athletes must consume 200-300 calories at least two hours before a race, and another 200 calories in the ten minutes prior to the event. This intake can be accommodated with:

- Hard boiled Eggs
- Whole Peaches
- Green Tea
- Protein Meat

During the race or exercise period, it is important to consume calories and carbohydrates in one of the following forms:

- Sports Drink
- Carbohydrate Gels or Chews

Directly following the race, calories, carbohydrates and glucose will have to be reintroduced into the body to help the initial healing process, which can take place in the form of the following:

• Fruit & Fruit Juice Smoothie with Glucose and Protein Powders

• Water, Water & MORE WATER!

• Raisins or Bananas to increase Alkalinity

• Cantaloupe

Lunch or Short Term Meal Option

• Grilled, Baked or Roasted Chicken or Turkey Sandwich

• Herbed Potatoes

• Fresh, Raw Vegetables or Flash Cooked Asparagus, Zucchini or Squash

• Apples

Dinner or Long Term Meal Option

• Salmon, Tuna or Other High-Protein Fish

• Streamed Spinach or Kale

• Mixed Green Salad with Avocados, Strawberries and Orange Slices

During peak performance training and execution, the athlete's carbohydrate intake will reach sixty percent of total calories, which is incredibly different than the standard Paleolithic Diet practitioner, but necessary to their overall health and ability to compete.

The overall benefits of the Paleolithic Diet are clear, and can help transform your body into a fitter, trimmer version of your previous existence. Your hair, skin and appearance will all appear smoother, shinier and healthier, while your internal health will improve immensely.

When people eat an unhealthy diet for an extended period of time, the visceral fat that evolves because of the processed, high sodium fat intake collects directly around the organs. This means they have to work harder, at a consistent rate to do the same job they previously did with very little effort. This is when health issues become a factor. Because your organs are working overtime, your blood is pumping at an irregular rate, and is being forced to circulate, instead of being allowed to flow properly.

This can cause heart disease, high blood pressure, diabetes, and organ damage if it isn't reversed through weight loss and healthy eating.

In addition, extra weight and an unhealthy appearance can lead to depression, low self-esteem and social withdrawal. Each of these side effects can lead to anxiety, self-loathing and a negative attitude towards life and relationships.

Starting this diet now can help you begin feeling better, less bloated, and more active than ever before. Simply begin by tossing all of the unhealthy items in your home, and take a pledge to a new grocery list of healthy, Paleolithic Diet eating alternatives.

Once you get started, your body will begin to crave all of the nutritiously approved foods daily, and the process will become a seamless application of health and happiness.

As with any diet plan, it is just as important for you to remain positive about the experience as is it to practice it. Consider all of the great things you are going to gain from this new diet plan, including a smaller size and a boost in your overall appearance.

Your commitment to the plan is key, but you should allow yourself to be treated to something that isn't on the normal menu from time to time. Every couple weeks or so, replace your snack in a single day with something fun, like a small bag of popcorn, so you do not feel confined to the diet at all times.

Remember, if you get frustrated with the process, you are more likely to abandon it, so give yourself a bit of wiggle room from time to time, but DO NOT GO CRAZY with it. You certainly should not replace your usually delicious and nutritious lunch salad with a bucket of fried chicken. At no time, no matter which diet you are following, does that make any sense whatsoever.

That is what any diet plan is all about, making sense. No, you cannot eat cheeseburgers every day and expect to be healthy and thin -- no one can! But you can adapt completely healthy eating habits that do not ask you to starve yourself, or lock yourself in your home with home delivery meals, until you have lost the pounds you have always wanted to shed.

Instead, the Paleolithic Diet takes a realistic and healthy approach to transforming your body into a healthier, thinner you -- and in a significantly less amount of time.

What are you waiting for? Start compiling a list of the things you eat now, and start looking for options to put to the side in favor of a healthier Paleolithic dieting option. It will not take long to get used to the process, and you will be able to enjoy a menagerie of new foods as a result!

Closing Thoughts

Dieters around the world can lament their ups and downs with certain dieting programs, in addition to the number of versions they have tried over the years. The word diet in and of itself, carries a stigma that involves low-fat foods, and in very small portions, which makes the mere idea of beginning the process daunting.

At some point, mentioning the word "diet" to others began warranting responses of groans, and negative thoughts, which has led to people keeping their dieting choices to themselves.

When this happens, the dieter feels shamed or teased by others because of their choice to get healthy or to lose weight. Some people even go out of their way to order the worst menu item possible in front of the dieter, just to oppose the very idea.

A couple of things happen during these unsupportive stints a dieter encounters. First, the dieter's support group crumbles. Instead of being cheered on to champion a good cause of health and happiness, he or she is shamed into feeling bad about their decision.

This is typically the result of lunching with someone who has a low self-esteem, and refuses to allow anyone else to feel good about themselves in his or her company. Next, it may cause the dieter to abandon their healthy lunch choice, and pick something extreme to eat as a result.

This is always why so many diets fail. The other reason falls into the opposite side of the spectrum: The idea of practically starving yourself, or jarring your body with a trendy cleanse in an unhealthy and unrealistic attempt at losing weight.

Dieters need true answers to healthy eating, and a positive source of nutrition to counter their cravings throughout the day. Not fad options that can do more harm to the body than good, or provide short-term solutions to weight loss.

Dieting can be accomplished naturally, with positive results, allowing a better you to appear on the other side of its institution, thanks to the Paleolithic Diet, or "Paleo Diet".

Say goodbye to crazy shake concoctions, sub-standard meals delivered to your home, counting points or measuring your food. You no longer have to be a slave to your dieting routine, and this plan can prove it. You can simply enjoy every, single meal you eat while maintaining a healthy weight and energy level each day.

THE END

IF YOU ENJOYED THIS BOOK

YOU'RE SURE TO ENJOY THE BEST SELLERS BELOW

RECOMMENDED READS

Wheat Belly: Lose the Wheat, Lose the Weight, and Find Your Path Back To Health
By William Davis MD

Eat to Live: The Amazing Nutrient-Rich Program for Fast and Sustained Weight Loss
By Joel Fuhrman

The 100: Count ONLY Sugar Calories and Lose Up to 18 Lbs. in 2 Weeks
By Jorge Cruise

It Starts With Food: Discover the Whole30 and Change Your Life in Unexpected Ways
By Melissa Hartwig and Dallas Hartwig

About the Author

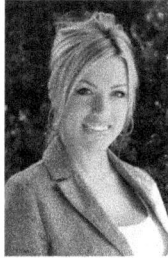

Mackenzie Jagger was born and raised in Baltimore, Maryland. Currently an event planner that recently turned 30 enjoys reading and writing about diet and fitness related subjects. She says her boyfriend is a bodybuilder and fitness "nut" and inspires her to be her best. She also loves to sing and dance.

Mackenzie Jagger's Author Page

https://www.amazon.com/author/mackenziejagger

Mackenzie Jagger's Website

http://TheFlatBellySolution.org

No part of this publication may be copied, reproduced in any format, by any means, electronic or otherwise, without prior consent from the copyright owner and publisher of this book.

www.ingramcontent.com/pod-product-compliance
Lightning Source LLC
Chambersburg PA
CBHW050556280326
41933CB00011B/1867